# How To Prevent West Nile Virus

I0096764

**Chapter 4** **31**

**Eliminating Mosquito Breeding Sites** **31**

Removing standing water 31

Maintaining swimming pools and ponds 33

Keeping gutters clean 35

**Chapter 5** **39**

**Protecting Your Home and Yard** **39**

Installing screens on windows and doors 39

Using mosquito traps 42

Hiring professional mosquito control services 44

**Chapter 6** **48**

**Traveling Safely** **48**

Tips for avoiding mosquito bites while traveling 48

Precautions to take in high-risk areas 50

Vaccination recommendations for travelers 53

**Chapter 7** **57**

**Recognizing and Treating West Nile Virus**     **57**

When to seek medical help     57

Treatment options for West Nile Virus     59

Long-term effects and complications of the virus     62

**Chapter 8Staying Informed and Prepared**     **66**

Monitoring local mosquito activity     66

Keeping up to date with public health warnings     68

Creating a West Nile Virus prevention plan     70

**Chapter 9**     **74**

**Conclusion**     **74**

Recap of key points     74

Maintaining a proactive approach to West Nile Virus prevention     75

Resources for further information and assistance     77

**Author Notes & Acknowledgments**     **80**

**Author Bio**     **82**

ISBN 978-1-998455-57-7 (Paperback)
ISBN 978-1-998455-58-4 (eBook)

Printed and bound in USA
Published by Loons Press

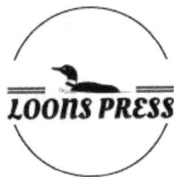

LOONS PRESS

# Table Of Contents

**Chapter 1**                                    **6**

**Understanding West Nile Virus**                **6**

What is West Nile Virus?                          6

History of West Nile Virus                        9

Symptoms of West Nile Virus                       11

**Chapter 2**                                    **15**

**Transmission and Risk Factors**                **15**

How is West Nile Virus transmitted?              15

Who is at risk for West Nile Virus?              18

Common misconceptions about West
Nile Virus                                        20

**Chapter 3**                                    **24**

**Preventing Mosquito Bites**                    **24**

Using insect repellent effectively              24

Wearing protective clothing                      26

Avoiding peak mosquito hours                     27

# How To Prevent West Nile Virus

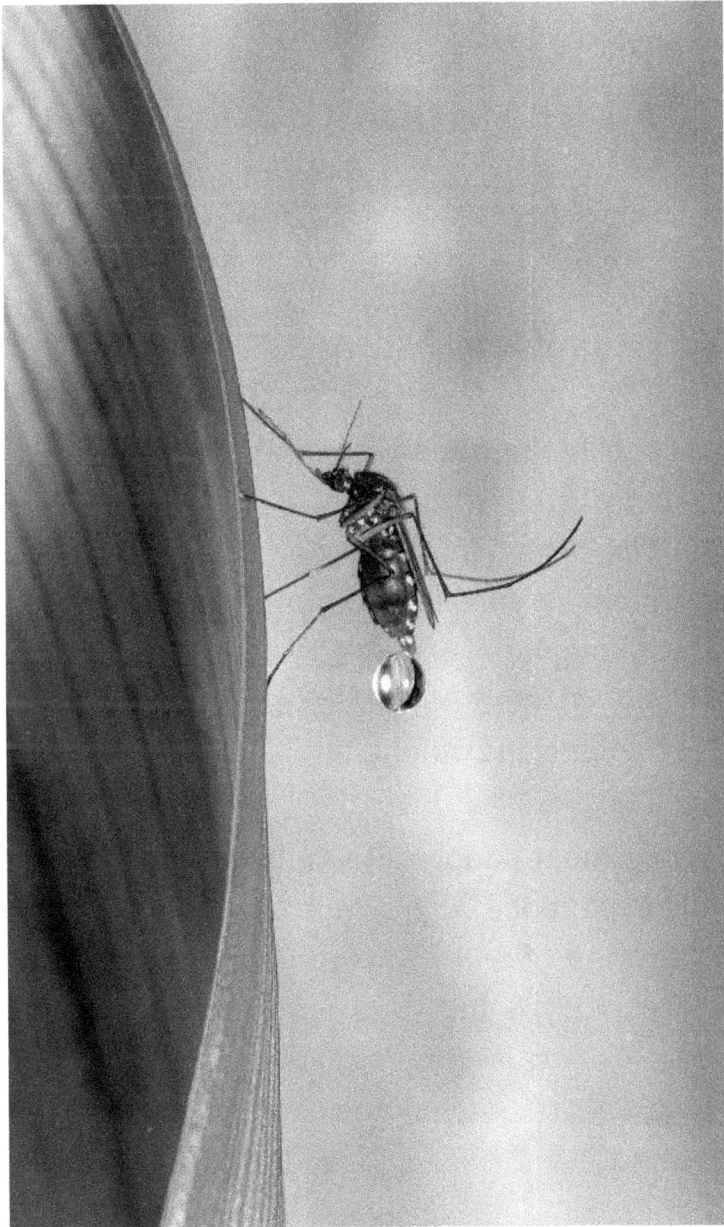

# Chapter 1

# Understanding West Nile Virus

## What is West Nile Virus?

West Nile Virus is a potentially serious illness that is primarily spread through the bites of infected mosquitoes. The virus is most commonly found in birds, which serve as the primary reservoir for the disease. Mosquitoes become infected with the virus by feeding on infected birds and can then transmit the virus to humans and other animals through their bites.

While most people infected with West Nile Virus will not experience any symptoms, some individuals may develop flu-like symptoms such as fever, headache, body aches, and fatigue. In severe cases, the virus can cause neurological symptoms such as encephalitis or meningitis, which can be life-threatening.

Preventing West Nile Virus is essential for protecting yourself and your loved ones from this potentially dangerous illness. One of the most effective ways to prevent West Nile Virus is to reduce your exposure to mosquitoes. This can be done by eliminating standing water around your home, as mosquitoes breed in stagnant water. Make sure to empty any containers that may collect water, such as flower pots, buckets, or bird baths. Additionally, use insect repellent when spending time outdoors, especially during peak mosquito activity times, such as dawn and dusk.

Another important step in preventing West Nile Virus is to protect yourself from mosquito bites. Wear long sleeves and pants when outdoors, especially in areas where mosquitoes are prevalent. Use mosquito nets over strollers or cribs when outside with young children, and consider installing screens on windows and doors to keep mosquitoes out of your home. It's also a good idea to avoid outdoor activities during peak mosquito activity times, or use mosquito repellent if you must be outside during these times.

# How To Prevent West Nile Virus

In addition to protecting yourself from mosquito bites, it's important to take steps to protect your home from mosquitoes as well. Make sure that window screens are in good repair and fit tightly to keep mosquitoes out of your home. Consider using mosquito-repellent candles or devices in outdoor living areas, and keep grass and shrubs trimmed to reduce mosquito breeding grounds.

If you have a swimming pool, make sure it is properly maintained and chlorinated to prevent mosquitoes from breeding in the water.

By taking these simple steps to prevent West Nile Virus, you can greatly reduce your risk of becoming infected with this potentially serious illness. Remember that prevention is key when it comes to protecting yourself and your loved ones from mosquito-borne diseases, so be proactive and take the necessary precautions to keep yourself safe. With a little effort and vigilance, you can enjoy the outdoors without worrying about the threat of West Nile Virus.

## History of West Nile Virus

The history of West Nile virus dates back to 1937 when it was first discovered in the West Nile district of Uganda. The virus is primarily transmitted to humans through the bite of infected mosquitoes, with certain species of birds acting as reservoir hosts. Over the years, the virus has spread to various parts of the world, including Europe, Asia, and the Americas. In 1999, the first cases of West Nile virus were reported in the United States, sparking widespread concern among health officials and the general public.

Since its introduction to the U.S., West Nile virus has become a significant public health concern, with thousands of cases reported each year. The virus can cause a range of symptoms, from mild flu-like illness to severe neurological complications. While most people infected with West Nile virus do not develop symptoms, those who do may experience fever, headache, body aches, and fatigue. In severe cases, the virus can lead to inflammation of the brain and spinal cord, resulting in long-term disability or even death.

# How To Prevent West Nile Virus

In response to the growing threat of West Nile virus, public health officials have implemented various strategies to prevent its spread. These include mosquito control measures, such as spraying insecticides and eliminating standing water where mosquitoes breed. In addition, individuals can protect themselves from mosquito bites by wearing long sleeves and pants, using insect repellent, and avoiding outdoor activities during peak mosquito hours.

By taking these simple precautions, people can reduce their risk of contracting West Nile virus and protect themselves and their loved ones from this potentially serious disease.

Despite the efforts to control West Nile virus, the virus continues to pose a threat to public health. As climate change and urbanization create more favorable conditions for mosquitoes to thrive, the risk of West Nile virus transmission is expected to increase. It is essential for individuals to stay informed about the latest developments in West Nile virus prevention and to take proactive measures to protect themselves.

By following the recommendations of public health officials and practicing good mosquito control habits, people can reduce their risk of contracting West Nile virus and stay healthy and safe.

## Symptoms of West Nile Virus

One of the key factors in protecting yourself from West Nile virus is being able to recognize the symptoms early on. Knowing what to look for can help you seek medical attention promptly and prevent any complications from arising. The symptoms of West Nile virus can vary from person to person, but there are some common signs to be aware of.

The most common symptom of West Nile virus is fever, which can range from mild to severe. Other symptoms may include headache, body aches, fatigue, and sometimes a skin rash. In severe cases, the virus can lead to a condition known as West Nile encephalitis, which can cause inflammation of the brain and spinal cord. This can result in symptoms such as confusion, muscle weakness, and even paralysis.

It is important to note that not everyone infected with the West Nile virus will develop symptoms. In fact, the majority of people who are infected will not experience any symptoms at all. However, for those who do develop symptoms, it is crucial to seek medical attention as soon as possible. Early detection and treatment can help prevent the virus from progressing to a more serious stage.

If you suspect that you may have been infected with the West Nile virus, it is important to consult with a healthcare provider for proper diagnosis and treatment. Your doctor may recommend a blood test to confirm the presence of the virus in your system. In the meantime, it is important to rest, stay hydrated, and take over-the-counter medications to help alleviate symptoms such as fever and body aches.

Preventing West Nile virus is the best course of action, but being able to recognize the symptoms early on is also crucial. By staying informed and knowing what to look for, you can protect yourself and your loved ones from the potential dangers of this mosquito-borne illness.

Remember, early detection is key in preventing the virus from causing serious complications. Stay vigilant and take proactive measures to safeguard your health.

# How To Prevent West Nile Virus

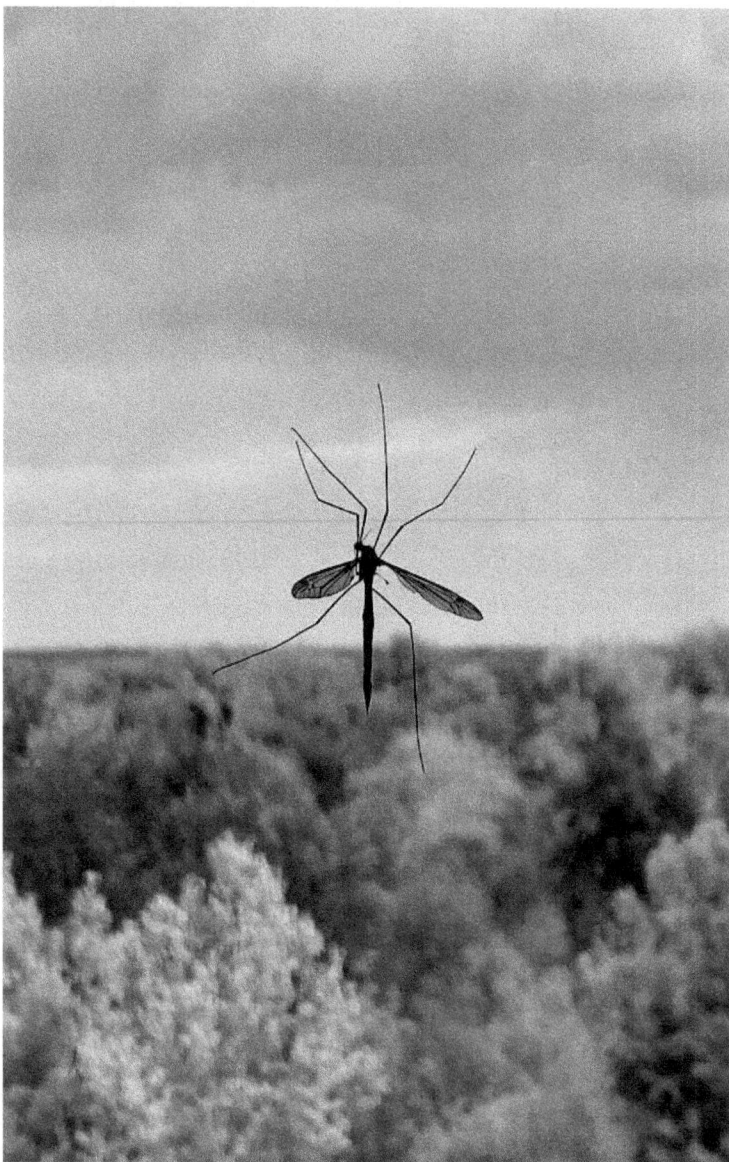

# Chapter 2

# Transmission and Risk Factors

## How is West Nile Virus transmitted?

West Nile Virus is primarily transmitted to humans through the bite of an infected mosquito. Mosquitoes become infected with the virus when they feed on infected birds, which serve as the primary reservoir for the virus. Once infected, mosquitoes can then transmit the virus to humans and other animals through their bites. It is important to note that not all mosquitoes carry the West Nile Virus, but it is still crucial to take precautions to avoid mosquito bites.

In addition to mosquito bites, West Nile Virus can also be transmitted through blood transfusions, organ transplants, and from mother to baby during pregnancy, childbirth, or breastfeeding.

While these modes of transmission are less common than mosquito bites, they are still important to be aware of, especially for individuals who may be at higher risk for severe complications from the virus. It is essential to follow proper safety measures and screening protocols to prevent the transmission of West Nile Virus through blood transfusions and organ transplants.

One of the key ways to prevent the transmission of West Nile Virus is to reduce exposure to mosquitoes. This can be done by wearing long sleeves and pants, using insect repellent, and avoiding outdoor activities during peak mosquito activity times, such as dawn and dusk.

Additionally, it is important to eliminate standing water around your home, as this is where mosquitoes breed. By taking these simple steps, you can greatly reduce your risk of being bitten by an infected mosquito and contracting the West Nile Virus.

It is also important to protect yourself and your family from other modes of transmission of West Nile Virus. If you are planning to donate blood or receive a blood transfusion, make sure to follow the necessary screening protocols to prevent the transmission of the virus. Similarly, if you are considering organ donation or transplantation, be sure to discuss the risks of West Nile Virus with your healthcare provider and follow their recommendations to minimize the risk of infection. By being proactive and informed, you can help protect yourself and your loved ones from the potential dangers of West Nile Virus.

Overall, understanding how West Nile Virus is transmitted is crucial for taking steps to prevent infection. By being aware of the primary modes of transmission, such as mosquito bites, blood transfusions, and organ transplants, you can make informed decisions to protect yourself and your family. By following simple prevention strategies, such as avoiding mosquito bites and taking precautions during blood transfusions and organ transplants, you can greatly reduce your risk of contracting the West Nile Virus and stay healthy and safe.

# Who is at risk for West Nile Virus?

West Nile Virus is a potentially serious illness that is spread through the bites of infected mosquitoes. While anyone can contract West Nile Virus, certain groups of people are at a higher risk than others. Understanding who is at risk, they can take necessary precautions to protect themselves from this disease.

Individuals with compromised immune systems, such as those undergoing chemotherapy or organ transplant recipients, are at an increased risk for developing severe symptoms of West Nile Virus. It is important for these individuals to take extra precautions to avoid mosquito bites, such as using insect repellent and wearing long sleeves and pants when outdoors.

Elderly individuals are also at a higher risk for developing severe symptoms of West Nile Virus. As we age, our immune systems may weaken, making us more susceptible to infections. It is important for older adults to take precautions to prevent mosquito bites, such as staying indoors during peak mosquito activity times.

Pregnant women are another group at risk for West Nile Virus. While the virus typically causes mild symptoms in pregnant women, it can lead to more serious complications for both the mother and the baby. Pregnant women should take precautions to avoid mosquito bites, such as using insect repellent and staying indoors during peak mosquito activity times.

Individuals who spend a lot of time outdoors, such as outdoor workers or athletes, are also at an increased risk for contracting West Nile Virus. These individuals should take precautions to prevent mosquito bites, such as wearing long sleeves and pants, using insect repellent, and avoiding outdoor activities during peak mosquito activity times.

By understanding who is at risk for West Nile Virus, individuals can take necessary precautions to protect themselves and their loved ones from this potentially serious illness.

## Common misconceptions about West Nile Virus

Common misconceptions about West Nile Virus can lead to unnecessary fear and confusion. One common misconception is that only certain groups of people are at risk for contracting the virus. In reality, anyone can become infected with West Nile Virus if they are bitten by an infected mosquito. This means that everyone, regardless of age or health status, should take precautions to protect themselves from mosquito bites.

Another common misconception is that West Nile Virus is only a concern during the warmer months. While it is true that mosquitoes are most active during the summer, West Nile Virus can still be a threat in the spring and fall. Mosquitoes can survive in cooler temperatures, so it is important to take precautions year-round to reduce your risk of contracting the virus.

Some people believe that using bug spray is enough to protect them from West Nile Virus. While bug spray is an important tool for preventing mosquito bites, it is not foolproof.

It is also important to wear long sleeves and pants when spending time outdoors, especially during dawn and dusk when mosquitoes are most active. Additionally, eliminating standing water around your home can help reduce mosquito breeding grounds.

Many people mistakenly believe that West Nile Virus is not a serious illness. While most people who become infected with the virus do not experience any symptoms, some individuals can develop severe complications, such as encephalitis or meningitis. These complications can be life-threatening, especially for older adults and individuals with weakened immune systems. It is crucial to take West Nile Virus seriously and take steps to protect yourself from mosquito bites.

Overall, it is important to educate yourself about the facts of West Nile Virus and take proactive steps to prevent infection. By understanding common misconceptions and taking practical measures to protect yourself, you can reduce your risk of contracting the virus and enjoy the outdoors safely.

# How To Prevent West Nile Virus

**Remember to follow guidelines from health authorities and take precautions year-round to protect yourself and your loved ones from West Nile Virus.**

# How To Prevent West Nile Virus

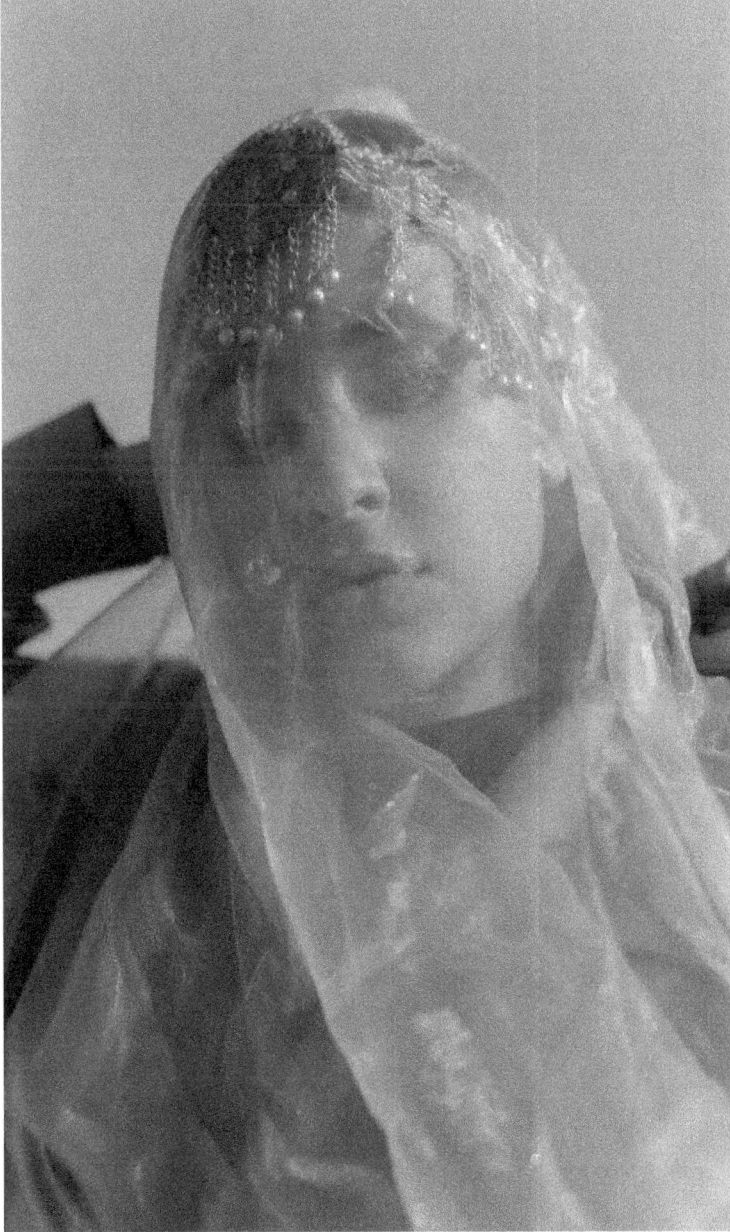

A Comprehensive Guide

# Chapter 3

# Preventing Mosquito Bites

## Using insect repellent effectively

Using insect repellent effectively is one of the most important steps you can take to protect yourself from West Nile virus. When choosing an insect repellent, it is important to look for one that contains DEET, picaridin, or oil of lemon eucalyptus, as these ingredients have been proven to be effective against mosquitoes that carry the virus. It is also important to apply the repellent properly, following the instructions on the label and reapplying as needed.

One common mistake people make when using insect repellent is not applying enough. To ensure maximum protection, be sure to apply a generous amount of repellent to all exposed skin. Remember to also apply repellent to clothing, as mosquitoes can bite through thin fabric. Additionally, be sure to reapply the repellent every few hours, especially if you are sweating or swimming.

It is also important to use insect repellent in conjunction with other preventive measures, such as wearing long sleeves and pants, using mosquito nets, and eliminating standing water around your home. By combining these strategies, you can greatly reduce your risk of contracting West Nile virus. Remember, mosquitoes are most active during dawn and dusk, so be especially vigilant during these times.

When using insect repellent on children, it is important to follow the recommendations on the product label. In general, it is safe to use repellent with up to 30% DEET on children over two months old, but be sure to avoid applying it to their hands, eyes, and mouths. For younger children, consider using clothing treated with permethrin or using a mosquito net over their stroller or crib.

By using insect repellent and in conjunction with other preventive measures, you can greatly reduce your risk of contracting West Nile virus. Remember to always read and follow the instructions on the product label, and to reapply the repellent as needed. By taking these simple steps, you can protect yourself and your loved ones from this potentially dangerous virus.

## Wearing protective clothing

Wearing protective clothing is an essential part of preventing West Nile virus. By covering up exposed skin, you can significantly reduce your risk of getting bitten by infected mosquitoes. When spending time outdoors, especially during peak mosquito activity times such as dawn and dusk, it is important to wear long sleeves, long pants, and closed-toe shoes. Additionally, wearing light-colored clothing can help deter mosquitoes as they are attracted to dark colors.

It is also recommended to wear clothing that is treated with insect repellent or to apply insect repellent directly to your skin. Look for repellents that contain DEET, picaridin, or oil of lemon eucalyptus for the most effective protection against mosquitoes. Be sure to follow the instructions on the product label and reapply as needed, especially if you are sweating or swimming.

When choosing your protective clothing, consider the thickness of the fabric. Thicker materials such as denim or canvas can provide an added barrier between your skin and mosquitoes.

Avoid wearing clothing made of thin, lightweight fabrics that mosquitoes can easily bite through. It is also a good idea to tuck your pants into your socks or wear socks over your pants to further prevent mosquito bites.

In addition to wearing protective clothing, it is important to take other precautions to prevent West Nile virus. This includes eliminating standing water around your home where mosquitoes can breed, using screens on windows and doors to keep mosquitoes out, and using mosquito netting over sleeping areas if you are camping or traveling to areas with high mosquito activity. By combining these strategies with wearing protective clothing, you can reduce your risk of contracting West Nile virus and enjoy the outdoors safely.

## Avoiding peak mosquito hours

Mosquitoes are most active during certain times of the day, known as peak mosquito hours. To avoid getting bitten and potentially contracting West Nile virus, it is important to be aware of when these peak hours occur.

# How To Prevent West Nile Virus

Typically, mosquitoes are most active during the early morning and evening hours, around dawn and dusk. By taking precautions during these times, you can greatly reduce your risk of being bitten.

One way to avoid peak mosquito hours is to plan your outdoor activities accordingly. If possible, try to schedule your outdoor activities for times when mosquitoes are less active, such as during the middle of the day. If you must be outdoors during peak mosquito hours, be sure to take extra precautions to protect yourself from mosquito bites. This may include wearing long sleeves and pants, using insect repellent, and avoiding areas where mosquitoes are known to be prevalent.

Another way to avoid peak mosquito hours is to make your living environment less attractive to mosquitoes. Mosquitoes are drawn to standing water, so be sure to eliminate any sources of standing water around your home, such as birdbaths, clogged gutters, and flower pots. By reducing the number of breeding sites for mosquitoes, you can help lower the mosquito population in your area and reduce your risk of being bitten.

In addition to avoiding peak mosquito hours, it is also important to take steps to protect yourself from mosquito bites at all times. This may include using insect repellent when outdoors, wearing protective clothing, and using screens on windows and doors to keep mosquitoes out of your home. By being proactive and taking these precautions, you can greatly reduce your risk of contracting West Nile virus.

In conclusion, avoiding peak mosquito hours is an important step in preventing West Nile virus. By being aware of when mosquitoes are most active and taking precautions to protect yourself during these times, you can greatly reduce your risk of being bitten. Additionally, by making your living environment less attractive to mosquitoes and taking steps to protect yourself from mosquito bites at all times, you can further lower your risk of contracting this potentially serious illness. Remember, prevention is key when it comes to protecting yourself from West Nile virus.

# How To Prevent West Nile Virus

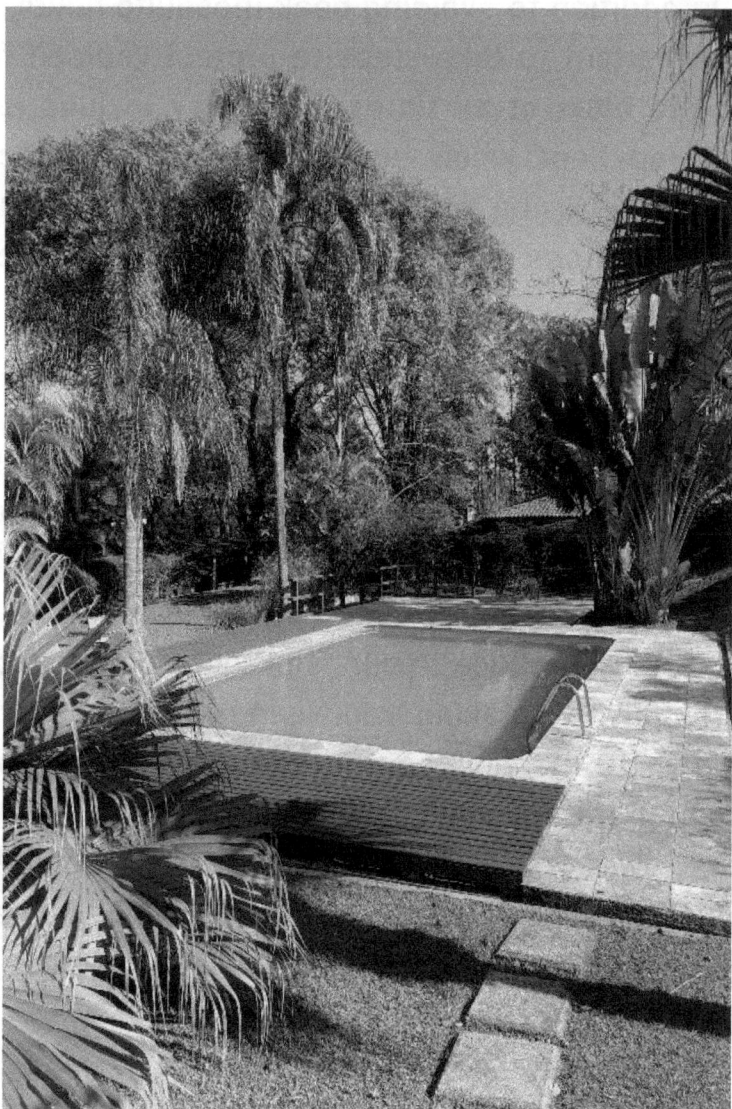

A Comprehensive Guide

# Chapter 4

# Eliminating Mosquito Breeding Sites

## Removing standing water

Standing water is a breeding ground for mosquitoes, which are carriers of the West Nile virus. Removing standing water from your property is one of the most effective ways to prevent the spread of the virus. Mosquitoes lay their eggs in standing water, and the larvae develop into adult mosquitoes within a matter of days. By eliminating standing water, you can significantly reduce the mosquito population in your area and lower your risk of contracting West Nile virus.

To effectively remove standing water from your property, start by checking for any containers that may collect water, such as buckets, flower pots, and bird baths. Empty these containers regularly to prevent mosquitoes from laying their eggs in them. You should also make sure that your gutters are clean and free of debris, as clogged gutters can create pools of standing water.

Additionally, check for any areas of poor drainage in your yard and address them to prevent water from accumulating.

Another important step in removing standing water is to properly maintain your swimming pool or hot tub. Make sure that the water is properly chlorinated and that the pool cover is free of standing water. If you have a decorative pond or water feature in your yard, consider adding aerators or pumps to keep the water circulating and prevent mosquito breeding. It is also important to regularly check for leaks or cracks in your plumbing that may lead to standing water.

In addition to removing standing water from your property, you can also take steps to prevent mosquitoes from entering your home. Make sure that your doors and windows have screens that are in good condition and free of holes. Consider using mosquito netting over beds and cribs, especially for infants and young children. You can also use mosquito repellent when spending time outdoors, especially during peak mosquito activity times, such as dawn and dusk.

By taking proactive steps to remove standing water from your property and prevent mosquitoes from entering your home, you can significantly reduce your risk of contracting West Nile virus. These simple and practical solutions can help protect you and your family from this potentially serious illness. Remember that prevention is key when it comes to West Nile virus, so be diligent in your efforts to eliminate standing water and reduce your exposure to mosquitoes.

## Maintaining swimming pools and ponds

Maintaining swimming pools and ponds is an essential part of preventing the spread of West Nile virus. Stagnant water in these areas can serve as breeding grounds for mosquitoes, which are carriers of the virus. By following a few simple maintenance tips, you can help reduce the risk of mosquito breeding and protect yourself and your family from West Nile virus.

First and foremost, it is important to keep your swimming pool clean and properly chlorinated. Mosquitoes are attracted to standing water, so maintaining a clean pool will help deter them from breeding in your backyard. Regularly check the chlorine levels and pH balance of your pool to ensure that it is safe for swimming and inhospitable to mosquitoes.

In addition to keeping your swimming pool clean, it is also important to maintain any ponds or water features on your property. Mosquitoes can breed in even small amounts of standing water, so be sure to regularly check and clean out any ponds or bird baths. Consider adding mosquito larvae-eating fish to your pond to help control mosquito populations naturally.

Another important step in maintaining swimming pools and ponds is to regularly inspect and repair any leaks or cracks that could lead to standing water. Mosquitoes only need a small amount of water to breed, so even a small leak in your pool or pond can provide an ideal breeding ground for these pests. By keeping your water features well-maintained, you can reduce the risk of mosquito breeding on your property.

Finally, consider adding mosquito-repelling plants around your swimming pool and pond area. Plants such as citronella, lavender, and marigolds are known to naturally repel mosquitoes and can help create a barrier between your outdoor living spaces and these pests. By taking a proactive approach to maintaining your swimming pools and ponds, you can help prevent the spread of West Nile virus and enjoy a safer and more enjoyable outdoor environment.

## Keeping gutters clean

One of the most effective ways to prevent the spread of West Nile virus is by keeping your gutters clean. Gutters that are clogged with leaves, debris, and standing water can become breeding grounds for mosquitoes, which are known carriers of the virus. By regularly cleaning your gutters and ensuring that they are free of any obstructions, you can significantly reduce the risk of mosquitoes breeding near your home.

To keep your gutters clean, it is important to perform regular maintenance throughout the year. Start by removing any leaves, twigs, and other debris that may have accumulated in your gutters. This can be done using a ladder and a pair of gloves to scoop out the debris by hand. It is also helpful to use a leaf blower or a pressure washer to flush out any remaining debris and ensure that the gutters are clear.

In addition to removing debris, it is essential to check for any signs of standing water in your gutters. Standing water is a prime breeding ground for mosquitoes, so it is important to ensure that your gutters are draining properly. If you notice any standing water, it may be necessary to adjust the slope of your gutters or install gutter guards to prevent water from pooling.

Another important step in keeping your gutters clean is to trim back any overhanging branches or vegetation that may be contributing to the clogging of your gutters. Branches that hang over your roof can deposit leaves and debris into your gutters, so it is important to regularly trim them back to prevent blockages.

By maintaining a clear path for water to flow through your gutters, you can help prevent the buildup of standing water and reduce the risk of mosquitoes breeding near your home.

By following these simple tips for keeping your gutters clean, you can help protect yourself and your family from the threat of West Nile virus. Regular maintenance of your gutters is an important step in preventing the spread of the virus, as it can help eliminate potential breeding grounds for mosquitoes. By taking the time to clean your gutters and ensure that they are free of obstructions, you can help reduce the risk of West Nile virus and keep your home safe and healthy.

# How To Prevent West Nile Virus

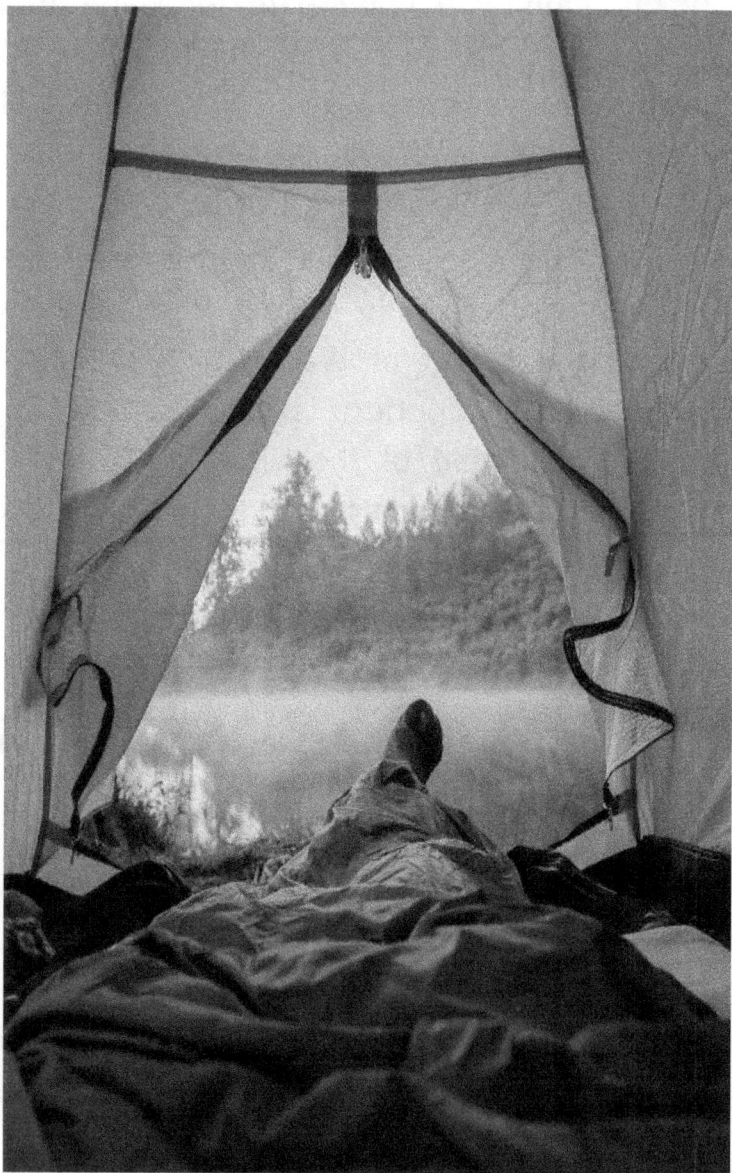

# Chapter 5

# Protecting Your Home and Yard

## Installing screens on windows and doors

Installing screens on windows and doors is a crucial step in protecting yourself from the threat of West Nile virus. Mosquitoes are the primary carriers of the virus, and they can easily enter your home through openings in windows and doors. By installing screens on all windows and doors, you can create a barrier that prevents mosquitoes from entering your living space. This simple yet effective measure can go a long way in reducing your risk of contracting West Nile virus.

When installing screens on windows and doors, it is important to choose high-quality materials that are durable and long-lasting. Look for screens that are made of strong mesh material that can withstand the wear and tear of daily use.

It is also important to ensure that the screens are properly fitted to each window and door, with no gaps or holes that mosquitoes could potentially squeeze through. Additionally, consider installing screens on all windows and doors in your home, including those in basements and attics, to provide comprehensive protection against mosquitoes.

In addition to installing screens on windows and doors, it is also important to regularly inspect and maintain them to ensure they are in good condition. Check for any tears or holes in the screens and promptly repair or replace them as needed. It is also a good idea to clean the screens regularly to remove any debris or dirt that could potentially clog the mesh and reduce its effectiveness in keeping mosquitoes out.

By taking these simple steps, you can ensure that your screens provide optimal protection against mosquitoes and reduce your risk of exposure to West Nile virus.

Another important consideration when installing screens on windows and doors is to make sure they are properly secured. Use sturdy frames and hardware to attach the screens to your windows and doors securely, ensuring that they cannot be easily dislodged by strong winds or other external forces. Additionally, consider adding weather-stripping or sealant around the edges of the screens to further prevent mosquitoes from finding their way into your home. By taking these extra precautions, you can enhance the effectiveness of your screens in keeping mosquitoes out and protecting yourself from West Nile virus.

In conclusion, installing screens on windows and doors is a simple yet effective way to protect yourself from the threat of West Nile virus. By choosing high-quality materials, properly fitting and maintaining the screens, and ensuring they are securely attached, you can create a strong barrier against mosquitoes entering your home. By taking these proactive measures, you can significantly reduce your risk of exposure to West Nile virus and enjoy peace of mind knowing that you are taking steps to protect yourself and your loved ones from this potentially dangerous disease.

## Using mosquito traps

Mosquito traps are a valuable tool in the fight against West Nile virus. These traps work by attracting and capturing mosquitoes, thereby reducing the overall mosquito population in an area. By using mosquito traps, you can significantly decrease your risk of being bitten by an infected mosquito and contracting the virus.

There are several different types of mosquito traps available on the market, each with its own unique features and benefits. One popular type of mosquito trap is the propane-powered trap, which releases carbon dioxide to attract mosquitoes. Another option is the electric trap, which uses a light source to lure mosquitoes and then traps them using a fan or adhesive pad. It is important to choose a trap that is suitable for your specific needs and budget.

When using mosquito traps, it is essential to place them in strategic locations around your property. Mosquitoes are attracted to areas with standing water, so be sure to place your traps near ponds, birdbaths, and other potential breeding grounds.

Additionally, consider placing traps near outdoor seating areas or other areas where you spend time outdoors to maximize their effectiveness.

In addition to using mosquito traps, there are several other steps you can take to protect yourself from West Nile virus. These include wearing long sleeves and pants when outdoors, using insect repellent containing DEET, and ensuring that your home is properly screened to keep mosquitoes out. By combining these preventative measures with the use of mosquito traps, you can significantly reduce your risk of contracting West Nile virus.

In conclusion, mosquito traps are a valuable tool in the fight against West Nile virus. By using traps in conjunction with other preventative measures, you can greatly reduce your risk of being bitten by an infected mosquito. Remember to choose a trap that suits your needs, place it strategically around your property, and take additional steps to protect yourself from mosquito bites. By taking these proactive steps, you can enjoy the outdoors with peace of mind and reduce your risk of contracting West Nile virus.

## Hiring professional mosquito control services

One of the most effective ways to prevent West Nile virus is to hire professional mosquito control services. These services are specifically designed to target and eliminate mosquitoes that may be carrying the virus. By hiring professionals, you can ensure that your property is properly treated and protected from these disease-carrying pests.

Professional mosquito control services use a variety of methods to effectively reduce mosquito populations. This may include treating standing water sources where mosquitoes breed, applying larvicides to kill mosquito larvae, and using adulticides to kill adult mosquitoes. By utilizing these techniques, professionals can significantly reduce the number of mosquitoes on your property and lower your risk of contracting West Nile virus.

When hiring professional mosquito control services, it is important to choose a reputable company with experience in mosquito control. Look for companies that are licensed and insured, and ask for references from satisfied customers. Additionally, be sure to inquire about the specific methods and products they use for mosquito control, and make sure they are safe for humans and pets.

In addition to hiring professional mosquito control services, there are other steps you can take to prevent West Nile virus. This includes wearing long sleeves and pants when outdoors, using insect repellent with DEET, and installing screens on windows and doors to keep mosquitoes out of your home.

By combining these preventative measures with professional mosquito control services, you can greatly reduce your risk of contracting West Nile virus.

Overall, hiring professional mosquito control services is an essential part of protecting yourself from West Nile virus. By taking proactive steps to eliminate mosquitoes from your property, you can greatly reduce your risk of exposure to this dangerous virus. Remember to choose a reputable company with experience in mosquito control, and be sure to follow all recommended preventative measures to keep yourself and your loved ones safe.

# How To Prevent West Nile Virus

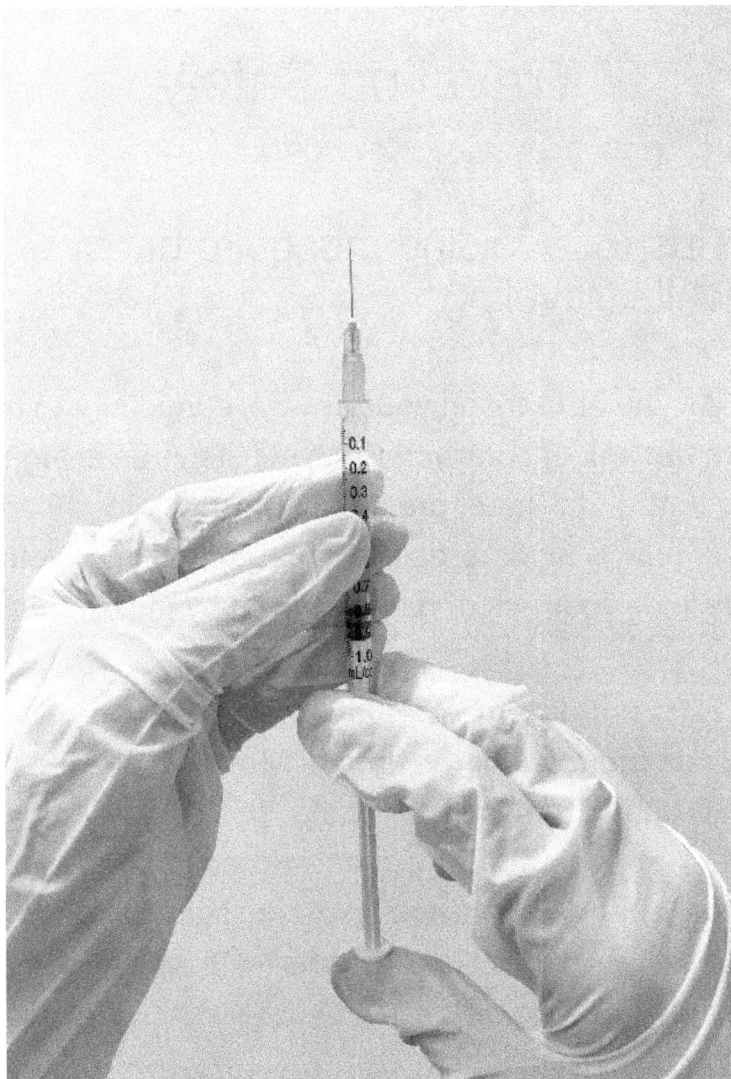

# Chapter 6

# Traveling Safely

## Tips for avoiding mosquito bites while traveling

As you embark on your travels, especially to areas where the risk of contracting West Nile virus is higher, it is essential to take precautions to avoid mosquito bites. Here are some tips to help you protect yourself and reduce your risk of getting bitten by mosquitoes.

First and foremost, it is important to be aware of peak mosquito activity times. Mosquitoes are most active during dawn and dusk, so try to limit your outdoor activities during these times. If you must be outside during these hours, make sure to wear long sleeves and pants to cover your skin and reduce the chances of getting bitten.

Another effective way to prevent mosquito bites while traveling is to use insect repellent. Look for repellents that contain DEET, picaridin, or oil of lemon eucalyptus, as these have been proven to be effective in repelling mosquitoes. Be sure to apply the repellent to all exposed areas of skin, and reapply as needed according to the instructions on the product label.

In addition to using insect repellent, consider wearing light-colored clothing. Mosquitoes are attracted to dark colors, so wearing light-colored clothing can help make you less appealing to them. You may also want to consider treating your clothing with permethrin, an insect repellent that can be applied to clothing to provide additional protection.

When staying in accommodations that are not air-conditioned or do not have screens on windows and doors, consider using a mosquito net. This can provide an extra layer of protection while you sleep and help prevent mosquito bites during the night. Make sure the net is properly secured and does not have any holes or tears that mosquitoes could enter through.

Lastly, be mindful of your surroundings and take steps to eliminate standing water where mosquitoes can breed. Empty any containers that collect water, such as buckets, flower pots, or bird baths. By reducing the presence of standing water around your accommodations, you can help reduce the mosquito population and lower your risk of getting bitten. By following these tips, you can protect yourself from mosquito bites while traveling and reduce your risk of contracting West Nile virus.

## Precautions to take in high-risk areas

Precautions to take in high-risk areas are crucial in minimizing the risk of contracting West Nile virus. When visiting areas known for high mosquito activity, it is important to take proactive measures to protect yourself from potential exposure. One of the first precautions to take is to wear long sleeves and pants to cover as much skin as possible. Mosquitoes are attracted to exposed skin, so minimizing their access to your skin can greatly reduce your risk of being bitten.

Additionally, using insect repellent containing DEET or picaridin is highly recommended when spending time outdoors in high-risk areas. These repellents are effective in deterring mosquitoes and can provide added protection against West Nile virus. It is important to apply the repellent to exposed skin and clothing to maximize its effectiveness. Reapplying the repellent as directed on the product label is also important to ensure continued protection.

Another precaution to take in high-risk areas is to avoid outdoor activities during peak mosquito hours, which are typically dawn and dusk. Mosquitoes are most active during these times, so staying indoors during these hours can significantly reduce your risk of being bitten. If you must be outside during peak mosquito hours, consider using mosquito netting or screens to create a barrier between yourself and mosquitoes.

In high-risk areas, it is also important to eliminate standing water around your home or property. Mosquitoes breed in standing water, so removing sources of standing water such as birdbaths, flowerpots, and clogged gutters can help reduce mosquito populations in your area. Additionally, using larvicides in areas where standing water cannot be eliminated can help control mosquito larvae and reduce the risk of mosquito-borne diseases like West Nile virus.

Overall, taking precautions in high-risk areas is essential in preventing West Nile virus. By following these practical solutions and incorporating them into your daily routine, you can greatly reduce your risk of contracting this potentially serious illness. Remember to stay informed about West Nile virus and take proactive measures to protect yourself and your loved ones from mosquito bites.

# Vaccination recommendations for travelers

Vaccination recommendations for travelers are an important aspect of preventing the spread of West Nile virus. When planning a trip to an area where the virus is prevalent, it is crucial to ensure that you are up to date on all recommended vaccinations. The Centers for Disease Control and Prevention (CDC) provides guidelines on which vaccines are necessary for specific regions, so be sure to consult with your healthcare provider before traveling.

In addition to routine vaccinations, there are specific vaccines that can protect against mosquito-borne illnesses like West Nile virus. The most common vaccine for travelers is the Japanese encephalitis vaccine, which can also provide some protection against other mosquito-borne diseases. It is important to get vaccinated at least a few weeks before your trip to ensure that your body has enough time to build up immunity.

For those planning to travel to areas where West Nile virus is endemic, it is recommended to take additional precautions to prevent mosquito bites. This includes using insect repellent with DEET, wearing long sleeves and pants, and staying indoors during peak mosquito activity times. In some cases, travelers may also consider taking prophylactic medications to prevent infection, especially if they are at high risk for complications from the virus.

It is important to note that there is currently no vaccine specifically for West Nile virus, so prevention through mosquito bite avoidance is key. However, staying up to date on all recommended vaccinations can help protect you from other mosquito-borne diseases that may be prevalent in the same areas. By taking the necessary precautions and staying informed about vaccination recommendations, travelers can reduce their risk of contracting West Nile virus and other illnesses while abroad.

In conclusion, vaccination recommendations for travelers are an essential part of preventing the spread of West Nile virus. By consulting with a healthcare provider and staying up to date on all recommended vaccines, travelers can ensure that they are protected against mosquito-borne diseases. In addition to vaccinations, taking preventative measures to avoid mosquito bites is crucial for staying safe while traveling to areas where West Nile virus is endemic. With proper planning and awareness, travelers can enjoy their trips without worrying about the risk of contracting this potentially serious illness.

# How To Prevent West Nile Virus

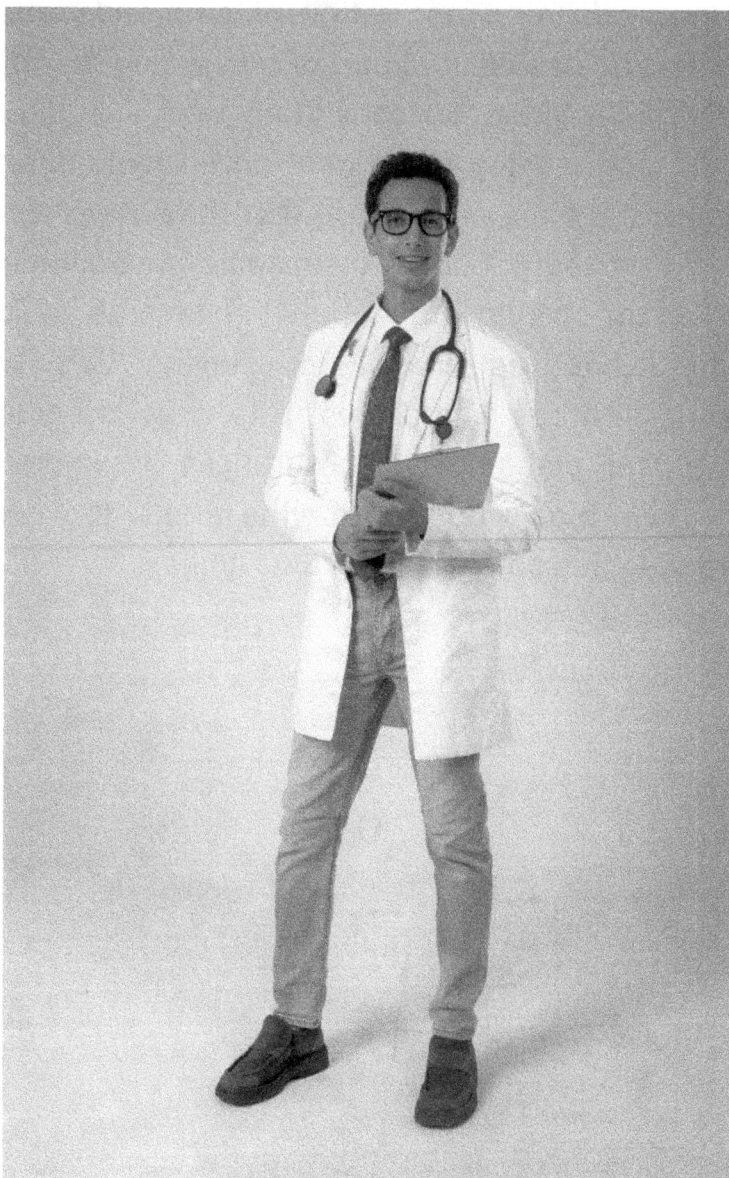

A Comprehensive Guide

# Chapter 7

# Recognizing and Treating West Nile Virus

## When to seek medical help

When it comes to protecting yourself from the West Nile virus, being proactive is key. While prevention methods are essential, it's also important to know when to seek medical help if you suspect you have been infected. Early detection and treatment can make a significant difference in your recovery, so it's crucial to be aware of the signs and symptoms of the virus.

One of the first signs of West Nile virus is flu-like symptoms, such as fever, headache, body aches, and fatigue. If you experience these symptoms after being bitten by a mosquito, it's important to seek medical help immediately. Other symptoms to watch out for include nausea, vomiting, diarrhea, and a rash. In severe cases, the virus can cause neurological symptoms such as confusion, muscle weakness, and seizures.

If you have been diagnosed with West Nile virus or suspect you may have it, it's important to follow your healthcare provider's recommendations for treatment. There is no specific antiviral medication for West Nile virus, so treatment focuses on managing symptoms and providing supportive care. This may include rest, hydration, and over-the-counter pain relievers to help alleviate fever and discomfort.

In some cases, West Nile virus can lead to severe complications, such as encephalitis or meningitis. These conditions can be life-threatening and require immediate medical attention. If you experience symptoms such as severe headache, neck stiffness, disorientation, or difficulty walking, seek medical help right away. Early intervention can help prevent further complications and improve your chances of a full recovery.

In conclusion, knowing when to seek medical help is crucial when it comes to protecting yourself from the West Nile virus. By being aware of the signs and symptoms of the virus and seeking prompt treatment if needed, you can minimize the impact of the infection on your health. Remember to follow prevention methods to reduce your risk of exposure to mosquitoes and stay informed about the latest developments in West Nile virus prevention and treatment.

## Treatment options for West Nile Virus

When it comes to treating West Nile Virus, there are several options available that can help alleviate symptoms and promote recovery. While there is no specific antiviral treatment for West Nile Virus, healthcare providers may recommend over-the-counter medications such as pain relievers and fever reducers to help manage symptoms like headache and body aches. In more severe cases, hospitalization may be necessary to provide supportive care such as intravenous fluids and respiratory support.

In addition to medical treatment, it is important for individuals with West Nile Virus to rest and stay hydrated to help their bodies fight off the infection. Getting plenty of rest can help boost the immune system and reduce the severity of symptoms. Drinking plenty of fluids, especially water, can help prevent dehydration and support the body's natural healing process.

For individuals experiencing neurological symptoms such as severe headache, confusion, or muscle weakness, it is important to seek medical attention immediately. These symptoms may indicate a more severe form of West Nile Virus that can lead to complications such as encephalitis or meningitis. Early detection and treatment can help prevent these complications and improve the chances of a full recovery.

In some cases, healthcare providers may recommend physical therapy or rehabilitation to help individuals recover from the effects of West Nile Virus. Physical therapy can help improve muscle strength and coordination, while occupational therapy can help individuals regain the ability to perform daily tasks. Speech therapy may also be recommended for individuals experiencing speech or swallowing difficulties.

Overall, the key to treating West Nile Virus is early detection and prompt medical intervention. By seeking medical attention at the first sign of symptoms and following the treatment recommendations of healthcare providers, individuals can increase their chances of a full recovery. It is also important to take steps to prevent mosquito bites in the future to reduce the risk of contracting West Nile Virus again.

## Long-term effects and complications of the virus

As we continue to learn more about the West Nile virus, it has become increasingly evident that the long-term effects and complications of the virus can be quite serious. For those who are concerned about the potential impact of the virus on their health, it is important to understand these potential long-term effects in order to take appropriate precautions and preventative measures.

One of the most common long-term effects of the West Nile virus is the development of neurological complications. This can include symptoms such as headaches, muscle weakness, and even paralysis in severe cases. These neurological complications can persist for months or even years after the initial infection, making it crucial to seek medical attention and monitor any changes in symptoms closely.

In addition to neurological complications, the virus can also lead to long-term issues with the immune system. This can result in a weakened immune response, making individuals more susceptible to other infections and illnesses. It is important for those who have been infected with the West Nile virus to take steps to support their immune system through a healthy diet, regular exercise, and adequate rest.

Another potential long-term complication of the West Nile virus is the development of chronic fatigue syndrome. This condition can cause persistent fatigue, muscle pain, and cognitive difficulties that can significantly impact daily life. It is important for individuals who have been infected with the virus to listen to their bodies and prioritize rest and self-care in order to manage these symptoms effectively.

Overall, the long-term effects and complications of the West Nile virus highlight the importance of taking preventative measures to protect yourself and your loved ones from infection. By following simple steps such as using insect repellent, wearing long sleeves and pants, and eliminating standing water around your home, you can significantly reduce your risk of contracting the virus and experiencing these potentially serious long-term effects. Stay informed, stay vigilant, and take proactive steps to safeguard your health and well-being.

# How To Prevent West Nile Virus

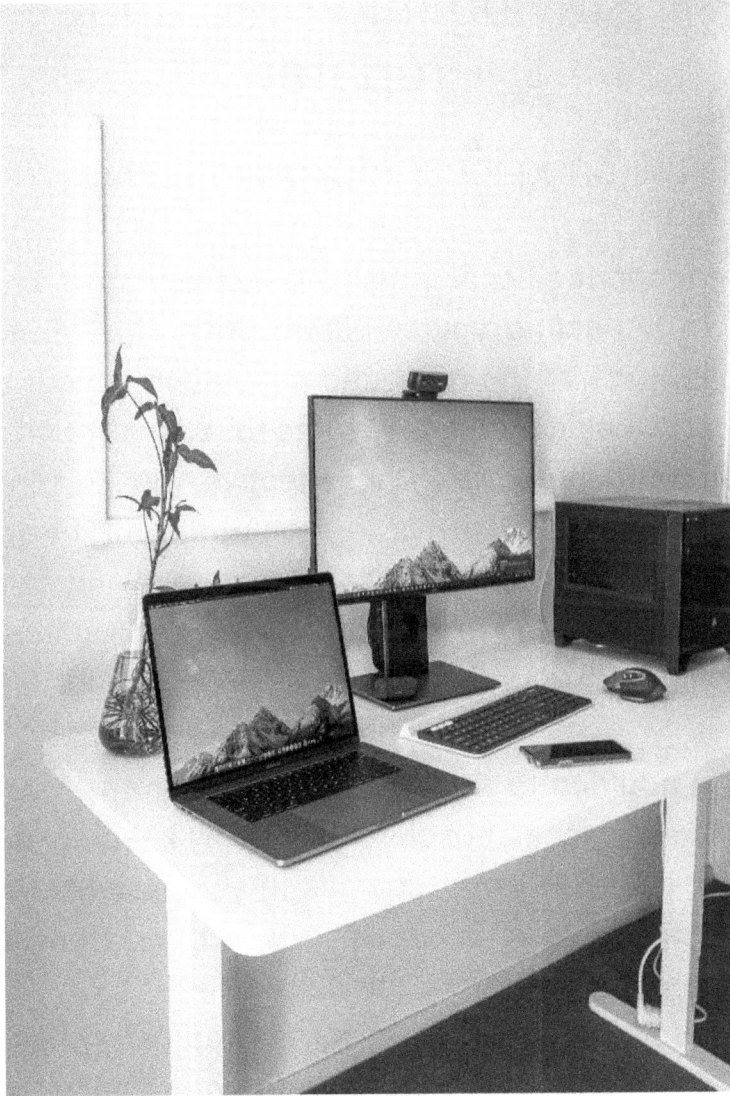

# Chapter 8
# Staying Informed and Prepared

## Monitoring local mosquito activity

Monitoring local mosquito activity is a crucial step in protecting yourself from West Nile virus. By keeping track of the mosquito population in your area, you can take proactive measures to reduce your risk of exposure to the virus. One effective way to monitor local mosquito activity is to set up mosquito traps in your yard. These traps attract mosquitoes and capture them, allowing you to track the number and species of mosquitoes in your area.

In addition to setting up mosquito traps, you can also monitor local mosquito activity by keeping an eye out for stagnant water sources in your neighborhood. Mosquitoes breed in standing water, so eliminating these breeding grounds can help reduce the mosquito population in your area. Be sure to regularly check for and empty any containers or areas of standing water, such as buckets, bird baths, and clogged gutters.

Another way to monitor local mosquito activity is to stay informed about mosquito control efforts in your community. Many local health departments and mosquito control agencies conduct surveillance and control activities to reduce the mosquito population and prevent the spread of West Nile virus. By staying informed about these efforts, you can better protect yourself and your family from mosquito-borne diseases.

It's also important to be aware of peak mosquito activity times in your area. Mosquitoes are most active during dawn and dusk, so it's best to avoid spending time outdoors during these times. If you do need to be outside during peak mosquito activity times, be sure to wear long sleeves and pants, use insect repellent, and take other precautions to prevent mosquito bites.

By monitoring local mosquito activity and taking proactive measures to reduce your risk of exposure to mosquitoes, you can protect yourself and your family from West Nile virus. Stay informed, eliminate breeding grounds, and take precautions to avoid mosquito bites to stay safe and healthy during mosquito season.

## Keeping up to date with public health warnings

Keeping up to date with public health warnings is crucial when it comes to protecting yourself from West Nile virus. Public health agencies regularly issue warnings and updates about the spread of the virus in different areas, as well as tips on how to prevent mosquito bites. By staying informed about the latest developments, you can take proactive measures to reduce your risk of contracting the virus.

One of the best ways to stay informed about public health warnings related to West Nile virus is to sign up for alerts from your local health department or the Centers for Disease Control and Prevention (CDC). These agencies often send out notifications about outbreaks, mosquito control efforts, and other important information that can help you protect yourself and your family. By subscribing to these alerts, you can stay ahead of the curve and make informed decisions about how to stay safe.

In addition to signing up for alerts, it's also important to regularly check the websites of public health agencies for updates on West Nile virus. These websites often have resources and information on how to prevent mosquito bites, as well as guidance on what to do if you suspect you may have been infected. By checking these websites regularly, you can ensure that you have the most up-to-date information on the virus and how to protect yourself.

Another important way to stay informed about public health warnings related to West Nile virus is to pay attention to local news reports. Local news outlets often cover outbreaks of the virus in specific areas, as well as tips on how to prevent mosquito bites. By staying tuned in to local news reports, you can get a sense of the current risk level in your area and take appropriate precautions to stay safe.

Overall, keeping up to date with public health warnings is essential for anyone concerned about West Nile virus.

By staying informed about the latest developments, signing up for alerts, checking agency websites, and following local news reports, you can take proactive steps to protect yourself and your loved ones from this potentially dangerous virus. By being vigilant and staying informed, you can reduce your risk of contracting West Nile virus and enjoy a healthier, safer summer.

## Creating a West Nile Virus prevention plan

Creating a West Nile Virus prevention plan is crucial for those who are concerned about protecting themselves from this potentially dangerous and deadly virus. By taking proactive steps to prevent mosquito bites and reduce the mosquito population in your area, you can significantly lower your risk of contracting West Nile Virus. In this subchapter, we will outline practical solutions and strategies for creating an effective prevention plan that will help keep you and your loved ones safe.

The first step in creating a West Nile Virus prevention plan is to focus on reducing your exposure to mosquitoes. This can be achieved by wearing long sleeves and pants when spending time outdoors, especially during the peak mosquito activity times of dawn and dusk. Additionally, using insect repellent containing DEET on exposed skin and clothing can provide added protection against mosquito bites. By taking these simple precautions, you can greatly reduce your risk of being bitten by an infected mosquito.

Another important aspect of a prevention plan is to eliminate standing water around your home, as this is where mosquitoes breed. By regularly emptying and cleaning out bird baths, flower pots, and other containers that collect water, you can help reduce the mosquito population in your area. Additionally, ensuring that your gutters are free of debris and properly draining can prevent water from pooling and becoming a breeding ground for mosquitoes. By taking these steps to eliminate breeding sites, you can significantly reduce the number of mosquitoes in your vicinity.

In addition to focusing on personal protection and reducing mosquito breeding sites, it is also important to consider community-wide efforts to prevent West Nile Virus. This can include working with local government agencies to implement mosquito control measures, such as spraying insecticides in areas where mosquitoes are particularly prevalent. By collaborating with your community and advocating for proactive mosquito control measures, you can help protect yourself and others from the threat of West Nile Virus.

In conclusion, creating a West Nile Virus prevention plan is essential for those who are concerned about protecting themselves from this potentially deadly virus. By focusing on reducing exposure to mosquitoes, eliminating breeding sites, and advocating for community-wide prevention efforts, you can significantly lower your risk of contracting West Nile Virus. By following the practical solutions outlined in this subchapter, you can take proactive steps to safeguard your health and well-being against this serious threat.

# How To Prevent West Nile Virus

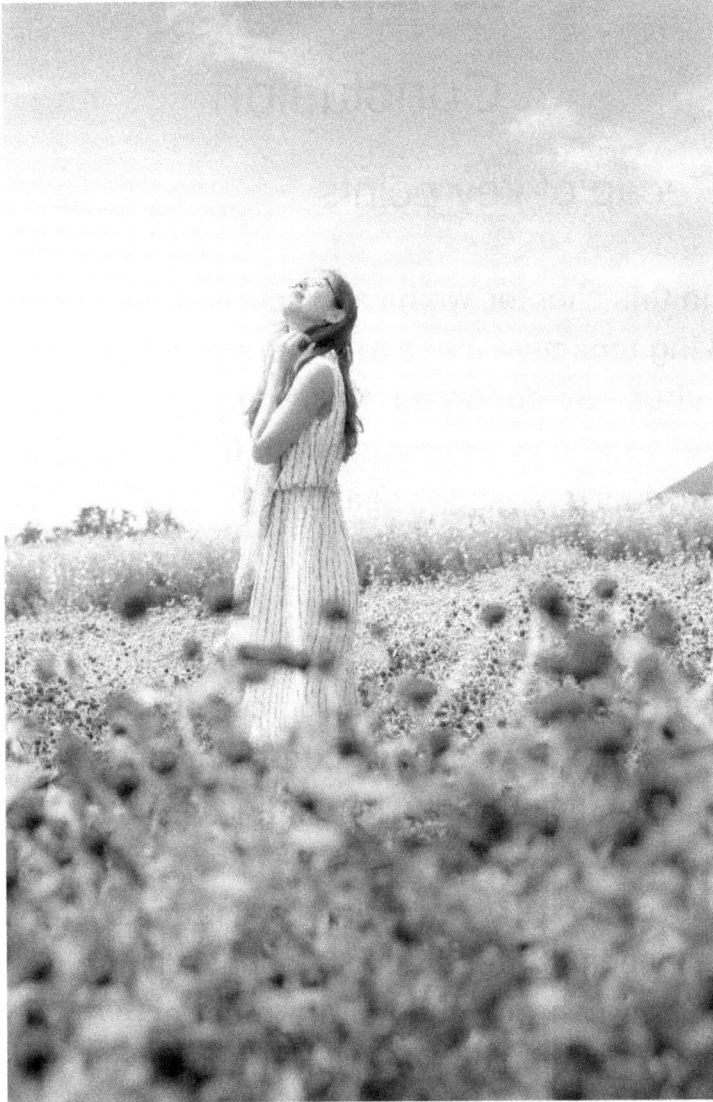

# Chapter 9

# Conclusion

## Recap of key points

In this chapter, we have discussed the importance of taking proactive steps to protect yourself from West Nile virus. By following these key points, you can reduce your risk of contracting the virus and stay healthy during mosquito season.

First and foremost, it is crucial to eliminate standing water around your home. Mosquitoes breed in stagnant water, so removing sources of standing water such as birdbaths, clogged gutters, and flower pots can help reduce the mosquito population in your area.

Secondly, it is important to use insect repellent when spending time outdoors, especially during dawn and dusk when mosquitoes are most active. Look for repellents containing DEET, picaridin, or oil of lemon eucalyptus, as these have been proven to be effective against mosquitoes carrying West Nile virus.

Additionally, wearing long sleeves and pants can provide an extra layer of protection against mosquito bites. While it may be tempting to wear shorts and t-shirts in hot weather, covering up can significantly reduce your risk of being bitten.

Finally, staying informed about West Nile virus activity in your area is key to protecting yourself and your loved ones. Be aware of any local advisories or warnings, and take appropriate precautions to avoid mosquito bites. By following these key points, you can reduce your risk of contracting West Nile virus and enjoy a safe and healthy summer season.

## Maintaining a proactive approach to West Nile Virus prevention

Maintaining a proactive approach to West Nile Virus prevention is essential for protecting yourself and your loved ones from this potentially dangerous disease. By taking simple yet effective measures, you can greatly reduce the risk of contracting the virus and minimize its impact on your health and well-being.

# How To Prevent West Nile Virus

One of the most important steps in preventing West Nile Virus is to eliminate standing water around your home. Mosquitoes, which are the primary carriers of the virus, breed in stagnant water, so by removing sources of standing water such as bird baths, flower pots, and clogged gutters, you can significantly reduce the mosquito population in your area.

Another key aspect of proactive prevention is to use insect repellent when spending time outdoors, especially during peak mosquito activity hours at dawn and dusk. Look for repellents containing DEET, picaridin, or oil of lemon eucalyptus, as these have been proven effective in keeping mosquitoes at bay. Be sure to follow the instructions on the product label for safe and effective use.

Wearing long-sleeved shirts and pants can also help to protect you from mosquito bites and reduce your risk of contracting West Nile Virus. Additionally, installing screens on windows and doors can prevent mosquitoes from entering your home and provide an extra layer of protection against bites.

Lastly, staying informed about West Nile Virus activity in your area is crucial for maintaining a proactive approach to prevention. By monitoring local news reports and public health alerts, you can stay ahead of potential outbreaks and take appropriate precautions to safeguard yourself and your community. Remember, prevention is key when it comes to protecting yourself from West Nile Virus, so be proactive and take the necessary steps to reduce your risk of exposure.

## Resources for further information and assistance

In this subchapter, we will provide you with a list of resources where you can find further information and assistance on how to prevent West Nile virus. These resources will help you stay informed and take proactive steps to protect yourself and your loved ones from this potentially dangerous disease.

One of the best resources for information on West Nile virus is the Centers for Disease Control and Prevention (CDC) website. The CDC provides up-to-date information on the latest outbreaks, prevention tips, and treatment options for West Nile virus. They also offer resources for healthcare professionals and local communities to help prevent the spread of the disease.

Another valuable resource is your local health department. They can provide you with information on local outbreaks, mosquito control programs, and tips for preventing mosquito bites. Your health department may also offer free or low-cost mosquito control services in your area, such as spraying for mosquitoes or distributing mosquito repellent to residents.

If you are looking for practical solutions to prevent West Nile virus, consider contacting a pest control company. They can help you identify and eliminate mosquito breeding grounds on your property, such as standing water in birdbaths, clogged gutters, or old tires. Pest control professionals can also recommend safe and effective mosquito repellents for outdoor use to protect yourself from bites.

Additionally, consider reaching out to local community organizations or environmental groups for assistance in preventing West Nile virus. Some groups may offer educational programs, community clean-up events, or resources for reducing mosquito populations in your area. By working together with your community, you can make a significant impact in reducing the risk of West Nile virus transmission.

Remember, knowledge is power when it comes to protecting yourself from West Nile virus. By utilizing these resources and taking proactive steps to prevent mosquito bites, you can significantly reduce your risk of contracting this potentially dangerous disease. Stay informed, stay vigilant, and take action to protect yourself and your loved ones from West Nile virus.

# Author Notes & Acknowledgments

First and foremost, I would like to express my deepest gratitude to the people who inspired and supported me throughout the journey of writing this book. This project would not have been possible without their unwavering belief in me and their invaluable contributions.

To my wife, thank you for your constant encouragement and understanding. Your love and support have been my anchor during the challenging times of researching and writing this book. Your belief in my ability to make a difference in people's lives has been my driving force.

I would also like to disclose that this book contains some renewed artificial intelligence-generated content. I really appreciate very recent technological innovation by outstanding scientists and of course our reader's understanding.

Lastly, I want to express my deepest gratitude to the readers of this book. I sincerely hope the strategies and methods outlined within these pages will provide you with the knowledge and tools needed to truly make your life much better. Your commitment to seeking any good solutions and willingness to explore multiple methods is commendable.

# Author Bio

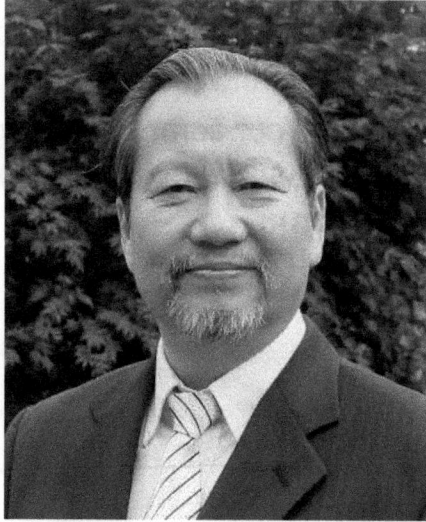

Johnson Wu earned his MD in 1982. With over 40 years of clinical experience, he has worked in hospitals in Zhejiang and Shanghai, China, as well as the Royal Marsden Hospital (part of Imperial College) in London, UK.

Upon the recommendation of Sir Aaron Klug, the president of The Royal Society and a Nobel Prize winner in Chemistry, Dr. Wu was honorably awarded a British Royal Society Fellowship. He has published medical books and articles in seven countries and currently practices medicine in Canada.

www.ingramcontent.com/pod-product-compliance
Lightning Source LLC
Chambersburg PA
CBHW060256030426
42335CB00014B/1720